COSMETIC INJECTION

EVERYTHING NEEDED TO KNOW

A Comprehensive Guide To Techniques, Safety, And Best Practices For Botox, Dermal Fillers, And Advanced Aesthetic Treatments

ROBERT LUGO

CHAPTER 1
Introduction And Overview

Cosmetic injections represent a significant aspect of modern aesthetic procedures, offering a range of treatments aimed at enhancing facial features, addressing aging signs, and improving overall appearance.

These injections utilize various substances, including neurotoxins, dermal fillers, and bio-stimulators, to achieve desired aesthetic outcomes.

The field of cosmetic injections has evolved considerably, driven by advancements in medical technology, increasing demand for non-surgical treatments, and a growing emphasis on natural-looking results.

Historical Perspective and Evolution

The history of cosmetic injections traces back to ancient civilizations, where natural substances like plant extracts and animal fats were used for facial enhancements.

However, the modern era of cosmetic injections began in the late 19th and early 20th centuries with the development of paraffin and silicone injections.

These early techniques laid the foundation for contemporary procedures, although they were associated with significant risks and complications.

The evolution of cosmetic injections accelerated in the mid-20th century with the introduction of collagen-based fillers, providing a safer and more reliable option for facial rejuvenation.

 Subsequent decades witnessed the emergence of hyaluronic acid fillers, botulinum toxin type A (Botox), and other innovative injectable, revolutionizing the field and expanding the treatment options available to patients.

Cosmetic injections play a crucial role in modern aesthetic medicine due to several key factors:

1. Non-Surgical Alternatives: Cosmetic injections offer non-surgical alternatives to traditional facial rejuvenation procedures, providing patients with minimally invasive options for enhancing their appearance without undergoing extensive surgery.

2. Targeted Treatments: Injectable procedures can target specific areas of concern, such as fine lines, wrinkles, volume loss, and facial asymmetry, allowing for precise and customized treatment plans tailored to each patient's unique aesthetic goals.

3. Natural-Looking Results: Advanced injectable techniques and formulations enable healthcare providers to achieve natural-looking results, preserving facial harmony and expression while addressing signs of aging and enhancing facial contours.

4.   Quick Recovery and Minimal Downtime: Compared to surgical interventions, cosmetic injections typically involve minimal downtime and quick recovery periods, allowing patients to resume their daily activities with minimal disruption.

5.   Versatility and Adaptability: The versatility of cosmetic injections extends beyond facial rejuvenation, with applications in lip augmentation, hand rejuvenation, neck and décolletage treatments, and non-surgical nose reshaping, among others.

This versatility enhances the appeal of injectable procedures for a wide range of aesthetic concerns.

6.   Patient Satisfaction and Confidence: Effective cosmetic injections can significantly impact patients' self-esteem and confidence by addressing visible signs of aging and enhancing facial features in a subtle yet noticeable manner.

Overall, cosmetic injections have become integral to the field of aesthetic medicine, offering safe, effective, and customizable solutions for patients seeking to enhance their natural beauty and rejuvenate their appearance without undergoing invasive surgery.

CHAPTER 2
Aesthetic Principles And Considerations

Aesthetic Principles in Cosmetic Injections

Cosmetic injections have revolutionized the field of aesthetic medicine by offering non-surgical solutions to enhance facial features and restore youthfulness.

Aesthetic principles guide practitioners in achieving harmonious and balanced results that align with the patient's desired outcomes and natural features. These principles encompass several key aspects that influence the success and satisfaction of cosmetic injection treatments.

Facial Symmetry and Proportions

Facial symmetry and proportions play a crucial role in aesthetic evaluations and treatment planning for cosmetic injections. Symmetry refers to the balanced arrangement of facial features on both sides of the face, while proportions involve the relative size and position of facial elements about each other. Achieving symmetry and ideal proportions enhances facial attractiveness and creates a more harmonious appearance.

Artistic Techniques for Natural-Looking Results

Artistic techniques in cosmetic injections involve the skillful application of injectables to achieve natural-looking results that enhance the patient's beauty without appearing overdone or artificial. This requires a deep understanding of facial anatomy, muscle dynamics, and product properties to create subtle enhancements that complement the patient's unique facial structure. Artistry in injection techniques involves precision, finesse, and a keen eye for detail to achieve optimal aesthetic outcomes.

Customizing Treatments for Individual Patients

Every patient is unique, with varying facial features, concerns, and aesthetic goals. Customizing treatments in cosmetic injections involves personalized assessment and planning to address each patient's specific needs and expectations.

This customization may include selecting the most suitable injectables, adjusting injection techniques, and tailoring treatment plans to achieve personalized and satisfying results for each individual.

Combining Methods to Get the Best Outcomes

Optimal results in cosmetic injections often require a combination of techniques to address multiple facial areas or concerns comprehensively. Combining techniques such as neuromodulator injections for dynamic wrinkles, dermal fillers for volume restoration, and collagen stimulators for long-term rejuvenation can yield synergistic effects and enhance overall aesthetic outcomes.

Strategic planning and expertise in combining techniques contribute to achieving natural-looking results with improved facial harmony and youthfulness.

aesthetic principles and considerations are fundamental to successful outcomes in cosmetic injections.

Understanding facial symmetry and proportions, applying artistic techniques for natural-looking results, customizing treatments for individual patients, and combining techniques when necessary are key factors in achieving optimal aesthetic results and patient satisfaction in the field of cosmetic injections.

CHAPTER 3

Types And Applications Of Cosmetic Injections

Types and Applications of Cosmetic Injections encompass a range of procedures and substances used to enhance facial aesthetics and address various concerns. Understanding these injections requires insight into their composition, mechanisms of action, and clinical applications.

Botulinum Toxin Injections, commonly known as Botox, are among the most popular cosmetic procedures globally. Botulinum toxin type A, derived from Clostridium botulinum bacteria, is used to temporarily paralyze muscles, reducing the appearance of wrinkles and fine lines.

Botox injections target dynamic wrinkles caused by repetitive facial expressions, such as frown lines, crow's feet, and forehead lines. The procedure involves precise injections into specific muscles, leading to a smoother, more youthful appearance.

Besides cosmetic use, Botox injections are also utilized in medical settings for conditions like migraines, excessive sweating (hyperhidrosis), and muscle spasms.

Dermal Fillers, including Hyaluronic Acid, Collagen, and other substances, are injectable treatments designed to add volume, contour, and rejuvenate the face. Hyaluronic acid fillers, such as Juvederm and Restylane, are popular for their ability to plump lips, soften facial lines, and restore lost volume in cheeks and under-eye areas. Collagen fillers, although less common now due to hyaluronic acid's widespread use, were historically used for similar purposes. Dermal fillers can also improve the appearance of scars and enhance facial symmetry.

Fat Transfer Injections involve harvesting fat from one part of the body (such as the abdomen or thighs) through liposuction, processing it, and injecting it into areas that require volume enhancement or contouring, like the face, breasts, or buttocks. This technique offers natural-looking results as the body's fat is used, reducing the risk of allergic reactions. Fat transfer injections are used to address hollowed cheeks, thin lips, and asymmetry, providing long-lasting results compared to some other fillers.

Platelet-rich plasma (PRP) Injections harness the body's natural healing abilities to rejuvenate the skin. PRP is obtained by drawing a small amount of the patient's blood, processing it to concentrate platelets and growth factors, and then injecting it back into targeted areas. PRP injections stimulate collagen production, improve skin texture, and can be used for facial rejuvenation, hair restoration, and scar revision. The growth factors in PRP promote tissue regeneration and help address signs of aging.

Neuromodulators and Neurotoxins refer to a class of substances that modulate nerve activity and muscle contractions.

Apart from Botox, other neuromodulators like Dysport and Xeomin are used for similar purposes, targeting facial muscles to reduce wrinkles and lines. These injections work by blocking signals between nerves and muscles, temporarily relaxing muscle contractions responsible for dynamic wrinkles.

Neuromodulators are commonly used for frown lines, crow's feet, and brow lifting, providing noticeable but natural-looking results.

Each type of cosmetic injection has specific indications, benefits, and considerations. Understanding their applications and potential outcomes is crucial for both practitioners and patients seeking cosmetic enhancements.

These injections, when performed by qualified professionals with proper technique and attention to individual needs, can significantly improve facial aesthetics and boost self-confidence.

CHAPTER 4

Preparation And Patient Assessment

In the realm of cosmetic injections, thorough preparation, and patient assessment are pivotal for ensuring safety, efficacy, and patient satisfaction. The process begins with a comprehensive patient assessment and consultation, where the practitioner gathers essential information to tailor the treatment plan to the individual's unique needs and goals.

This assessment encompasses several key aspects, including reviewing the patient's medical history, identifying contraindications, conducting the informed consent process, and adhering to pre-procedure protocols and guidelines.

Patient assessment and consultation are foundational steps that set the stage for a successful cosmetic injection procedure. During the initial consultation, the practitioner engages in open dialogue with the patient to understand their aesthetic concerns, desired outcomes, medical history, and any pre-existing conditions.

This dialogue fosters trust and transparency, enabling the practitioner to make informed recommendations and develop a personalized treatment plan.

A critical component of patient assessment is the review of medical history and identification of contraindications. This entails a detailed review of past medical conditions, surgeries, allergies, medications, and previous cosmetic procedures. Certain medical conditions and medications may contraindicate or require special considerations for cosmetic injections, necessitating careful evaluation and consultation with other healthcare providers when necessary.

The informed consent process is a fundamental aspect of ethical practice in cosmetic injections.

It involves providing patients with comprehensive information about the proposed treatment, including potential risks, benefits, alternatives, expected outcomes, and post-procedure care instructions. Informed consent ensures that patients have a thorough understanding of the procedure and actively participate in decision-making regarding their aesthetic journey.

Pre-procedure protocols and guidelines are established to optimize safety and procedural outcomes. These protocols may include pre-treatment assessments, skin preparation, anesthesia considerations, injection techniques, and post-procedure monitoring. Adhering to these guidelines minimizes risks, enhances patient comfort, and promotes optimal results.

Overall, thorough preparation and patient assessment are essential pillars of responsible and effective cosmetic injection practice.

By prioritizing patient safety, informed decision-making, and adherence to established protocols, practitioners can deliver exceptional aesthetic outcomes and ensure positive patient experiences.

CHAPTER 5
Injection Techniques And Precision

Injection techniques and precision in cosmetic procedures are critical aspects that demand a deep understanding of anatomy, physiology, and advanced procedural skills. The efficacy and safety of cosmetic injections rely heavily on the practitioner's ability to employ precise techniques tailored to specific anatomical areas.

In this comprehensive exploration, we delve into the intricate details of injection techniques, anatomical considerations, and strategies for managing patient comfort and pain.

Anatomy and Physiology Relevant to Injection Sites:

To master injection techniques, a solid grasp of the underlying anatomy and physiology of relevant injection sites is indispensable. Each area of the face and body presents unique anatomical structures such as muscles, nerves, blood vessels, and fat pads that influence injection outcomes.

Understanding the spatial relationships between these structures is paramount to avoid complications and achieve optimal aesthetic results.

The choice between using a needle or a cannula for cosmetic injections is a crucial decision that depends on factors such as the target area, desired outcome, patient comfort, and the practitioner's expertise.

Needles offer precision for precise placement in small or intricate areas, while cannulas are preferred for larger areas requiring broader product distribution with reduced trauma and bruising. Each method has its advantages and considerations, making it essential for practitioners to be proficient in both techniques for versatile and effective treatments.

Different facial and body areas require specific precision techniques to achieve desired aesthetic enhancements.

For instance, delicate areas like the lips demand meticulous injection placement to create natural-looking volume and contour, while deeper injections may be necessary for addressing volume loss in areas like the cheeks or temples.

Precision techniques also vary when targeting dynamic areas such as the forehead or crow's feet, where muscle movement influences injection outcomes.

Depth of Injection and Product Distribution:

The depth of injection plays a pivotal role in determining the spread and longevity of injected products. Understanding the ideal depth for each injection site ensures proper product distribution and avoids complications such as vascular compromise or uneven results.

Techniques such as serial puncture, fanning, and cross-hatching are employed to achieve even product distribution and enhance the overall aesthetic outcome.

Patient comfort and pain management are integral aspects of cosmetic injections that significantly impact the patient experience and treatment outcomes. Techniques such as topical anesthesia, nerve blocks, and the use of products with built-in anesthetics contribute to minimizing discomfort during injections.

Moreover, effective communication, a gentle approach, and a supportive environment help alleviate patient anxiety and enhance overall satisfaction with the procedure.

Mastering injection techniques and precision in cosmetic procedures requires a comprehensive understanding of anatomical nuances, proficiency in various injection methods, and a patient-centered approach to ensure optimal outcomes and patient satisfaction.

CHAPTER 6
Post-Procedure Care And Complications

Post-procedure care and complications are crucial aspects of cosmetic injections that require thorough understanding and management to ensure optimal outcomes for patients.

In this section, we delve into the immediate post-injection protocols, common reactions and their management, complications prevention, recognition, and treatment, as well as the importance of follow-up appointments and monitoring.

Immediate Post-Injection Protocols Immediately after receiving cosmetic injections, patients should adhere to specific protocols to promote healing and minimize potential complications.

These protocols often include:

1.   Rest and Recovery: Patients are advised to rest and avoid strenuous activities for a certain period following the injection.

This allows the injected substances to settle and reduces the risk of displacement or uneven distribution.

2.   Ice Application: Applying ice packs or cold compresses to the injection site can help reduce swelling and discomfort. However, patients should follow instructions regarding the duration and frequency of ice application to avoid skin damage.

3.   Avoiding Pressure: Patients should avoid putting pressure on the injection site, such as sleeping on the treated area or wearing tight clothing that could compress the injected material.

4.   Medication Compliance: If prescribed, patients should diligently follow the post-injection medication regimen, including pain

relievers or antibiotics, to manage any discomfort or prevent infections.

Common Reactions and Management Following cosmetic injections, patients may experience common reactions that are typically mild and temporary. These reactions may include:

1.   Swelling and Redness: It is common for patients to experience some degree of swelling and redness at the injection site. This usually resolves within a few days but can be managed with cold compresses and over-the-counter anti-inflammatory medications.

2.   Bruising: Bruising at the injection site may occur due to the injection process. Patients can manage bruising by applying arnica gel or cream, avoiding blood-thinning medications, and using camouflage makeup if desired.

3.   Tenderness and Sensitivity: The treated area may feel tender or sensitive to touch for a short period. Patients should avoid excessive

touching or rubbing of the area to prevent irritation.

4. Itching or Tingling: Some patients may experience mild itching or tingling sensations as the injected substance settles.

This is usually temporary and resolves on its own.

Complications: Prevention, Recognition, and Treatment While complications from cosmetic injections are rare, healthcare providers and patients should be aware of potential risks and take preventive measures. Key considerations include:

1. Infection Prevention: Strict adherence to aseptic techniques during the injection procedure and proper post-injection wound care can help prevent infections.

Patients should be educated on signs of infection, such as increased redness, swelling, warmth, or discharge, and instructed to seek medical attention if these symptoms occur.

2.   Allergic Reactions: Although uncommon, allergic reactions to injected substances can occur. Providers should inquire about patient allergies before treatment and be prepared to manage allergic reactions promptly with appropriate medications, such as antihistamines or epinephrine.

3.   Nerve Damage: Injection into or near nerve-rich areas carries a risk of nerve damage. Providers should have a thorough understanding of anatomy and injection techniques to minimize this risk. Patients should be informed about potential signs of nerve damage, such as numbness, tingling, or muscle weakness, and advised to report any unusual symptoms immediately.

4.   Vascular Complications: Injection into blood vessels can lead to vascular complications such as ischemia or necrosis. Providers should be skilled in recognizing vascular compromise and have protocols in place for prompt intervention, including aspirating to check for blood return

before injecting and knowing the anatomy of vascular structures in the treatment area.

Follow-Up Appointments and Monitoring Follow-up appointments are essential to assess the outcomes of cosmetic injections, address any concerns or complications, and make any necessary adjustments. Key aspects of follow-up appointments include:

1.   Assessment of Results: Providers evaluate the effectiveness of the injection treatment and discuss outcomes with the patient.

This may include comparing before-and-after photos, assessing symmetry and volume enhancement, and discussing patient satisfaction.

2.   Monitoring for Complications: Follow-up appointments allow providers to monitor for any delayed or emerging complications, such as infections, allergic reactions, or unusual healing patterns. Patients should be encouraged to report any new or worsening symptoms between appointments.

3. Touch-Up or Additional Treatments: Depending on the desired outcome and initial results, patients may benefit from touch-up injections or additional treatments to achieve optimal aesthetic results.

Providers can discuss these options during follow-up visits.

4. Long-Term Care: Patients should be educated on long-term care strategies to maintain the results of their cosmetic injections. This may include sun protection, skincare routines, lifestyle modifications, and regular follow-up appointments as needed.

Post-procedure care and complications management are integral aspects of cosmetic injections that require a collaborative approach between healthcare providers and patients.

By following appropriate protocols, monitoring for potential complications, and ensuring timely follow-up, patients can achieve safe and satisfactory outcomes from their cosmetic injection treatments.

CHAPTER 7
Advanced Techniques And Innovations

Advanced techniques and innovations in cosmetic injections have significantly transformed the landscape of aesthetic medicine. This evolution is driven by the constant pursuit of achieving more natural, long-lasting, and minimally invasive results. The field is expanding with novel approaches and technologies, enhancing both the efficacy and safety of procedures.

Understanding these advancements is crucial for practitioners aiming to provide state-of-the-art care and for patients seeking the best outcomes.

Advanced injection techniques have moved beyond traditional methods, incorporating new strategies to address specific aesthetic concerns. One such technique is the use of microcannulas, which are blunt-tipped instruments that allow for safer and more precise placement of injectable. Unlike needles, microcannulas minimize the risk of bruising and vascular damage, making them ideal for delicate areas such as under the eyes or around the lips. Their flexibility also enables practitioners to reach larger treatment areas with fewer entry points, resulting in a more comfortable experience for patients.

Another advanced technique involves the use of multi-layered injections. This approach considers the different layers of skin and subcutaneous tissue to achieve a more harmonious and natural look. For instance, deeper injections can provide structural support and volume, while more superficial injections can smooth out fine lines and wrinkles.

By strategically layering the injectable, practitioners can create a more balanced and aesthetically pleasing result that mimics the natural contours of the face.

Combination treatments have become a cornerstone of advanced cosmetic injection protocols.

By using a combination of different injectables, such as neurotoxins (e.g., Botox) and dermal fillers (e.g., hyaluronic acid-based products), practitioners can address multiple aesthetic concerns simultaneously.

For example, neurotoxins can relax dynamic wrinkles caused by muscle movement, while dermal fillers can restore volume and smooth out static wrinkles. This synergistic approach not only enhances the overall outcome but also extends the longevity of the results.

Combining injections with other aesthetic treatments further amplifies their effectiveness. For instance, pairing injectables with laser therapy can improve skin texture and tone, providing a more comprehensive rejuvenation.

Lasers can target pigmentation and stimulate collagen production, while injectable can restore volume and smoothness.

This holistic approach ensures that all aspects of aging are addressed, leading to a more youthful and refreshed appearance.

Advanced injection approaches also consider specific patient concerns and anatomical variations. Tailoring the treatment to the individual's unique facial structure and aesthetic goals is essential for optimal results. For instance, when addressing mid-face volume loss, practitioners may use a combination of deep injections to lift and support the cheek area and superficial injections to smooth out fine lines.

This precision ensures that the results are both natural and proportionate, avoiding the overfilled or unnatural look that can occur with less sophisticated techniques.

Integrating technology with injection procedures has opened new frontiers in cosmetic medicine.

Imaging technologies, such as ultrasound and three-dimensional imaging, allow practitioners to visualize the underlying structures of the face with remarkable clarity. This capability enhances the precision of injections, reducing the risk of complications and improving the accuracy of product placement.

 For example, ultrasound can help identify and avoid blood vessels, minimizing the risk of vascular occlusion, a rare but serious complication of dermal fillers.

Innovations in injection materials and delivery systems are also revolutionizing the field. New-generation dermal fillers are designed to provide more natural and longer-lasting results.

These fillers often incorporate advanced cross-linking technologies that increase their longevity and stability within the tissue. Additionally, bio-stimulatory fillers, such as those containing calcium hydroxylapatite or poly-L-lactic acid, not only provide immediate volume but also stimulate the body's collagen production, leading to longer-term improvements in skin quality and firmness.

The development of more sophisticated delivery systems has further enhanced the safety and efficacy of cosmetic injections.

For instance, needle-free injection devices use high-pressure jets to deliver hyaluronic acid or other substances into the skin without the use of needles. This technology reduces the risk of needle-related complications and improves patient comfort. Additionally, the advent of micro-dosing devices allows for precise control over the amount of product delivered, ensuring consistent and predictable results.

Another area of innovation is the use of combination products that integrate different active ingredients to achieve multiple effects. For example, some new formulations combine hyaluronic acid with lidocaine, a local anesthetic, to provide both volumization and pain relief in a single injection.

Other products may incorporate vitamins, peptides, or other bioactive compounds to enhance the overall skin health and rejuvenation effects of the treatment.

The application of regenerative medicine principles to cosmetic injections is an exciting frontier. Platelet-rich plasma (PRP) injections, for instance, harness the body's natural healing processes to improve skin texture and tone. PRP is derived from the patient's blood and contains a high concentration of growth factors that stimulate tissue regeneration and collagen production. When combined with dermal fillers or used on its own, PRP can enhance the overall rejuvenating effects of cosmetic treatments, providing a more holistic approach to anti-aging.

Research and development in the field of cosmetic injections continue to push the boundaries of what is possible. Ongoing studies are exploring the potential of stem cell-based therapies, which could offer even more profound and long-lasting rejuvenation effects.

These cutting-edge treatments aim to not only restore volume and smoothness but also to fundamentally improve the health and function of the skin at a cellular level.

The future of cosmetic injections is likely to see further integration of artificial intelligence (AI) and machine learning technologies.

AI-driven analysis can help practitioners develop highly personalized treatment plans by analyzing a vast array of data points, including facial anatomy, skin condition, and patient preferences.

This technology has the potential to optimize treatment outcomes and enhance patient satisfaction by ensuring that each intervention is precisely tailored to the individual's needs.

the advancements and innovations in cosmetic injection techniques are transforming the field of aesthetic medicine. By leveraging new technologies, combination treatments, and advanced materials, practitioners can achieve more natural, long-lasting, and comprehensive results.

These developments not only enhance aesthetic outcomes but also improve the safety and comfort of the procedures, making cosmetic injections a more attractive option for a broader range of patients. As the field continues to evolve, staying abreast of these innovations will be crucial for practitioners committed to providing the highest standard of care.

CHAPTER 8
Ethical And Legal Considerations

Ethical and legal considerations in cosmetic injections are multifaceted and require a thorough understanding of patient rights and responsibilities, ethical principles, legal regulations, and professional conduct. In the realm of aesthetic medicine, ensuring ethical practices and legal compliance is paramount to maintaining trust, safety, and efficacy in patient care.

Patient rights and responsibilities form the cornerstone of ethical practice in cosmetic injections. Patients have the right to be fully informed about the procedures they are considering, including the potential risks, benefits, and alternatives. This encompasses a comprehensive understanding of the nature of the injection, the expected outcomes, and any possible side effects or complications. Informed consent is a critical aspect, requiring that patients receive clear, understandable information and have the opportunity to ask questions and receive satisfactory answers before proceeding with any treatment. Moreover, patients have the right to receive care that respects their dignity, privacy, and confidentiality.

This means that practitioners must handle patient information with the utmost discretion and ensure that all interactions are conducted with respect for the patient's autonomy and personal circumstances.

Patients also have responsibilities in the context of cosmetic injections. They are expected to provide accurate and complete medical histories, including any previous procedures, allergies, and current medications.

This information is crucial for the practitioner to assess the suitability of the procedure and to plan appropriately for the patient's safety. Additionally, patients should adhere to pre- and post-procedure instructions provided by their healthcare providers to optimize outcomes and minimize the risk of complications. Following guidelines regarding medication use, lifestyle modifications, and follow-up appointments is essential for achieving the desired results and ensuring a smooth recovery process.

Ethical considerations in cosmetic injections involve a commitment to the principles of beneficence, non-maleficence, autonomy, and justice. Practitioners must prioritize the well-being of their patients, striving to achieve positive outcomes while minimizing harm.

This includes using evidence-based practices and adhering to safety protocols to reduce the risk of adverse effects. Non-maleficence, or "not harm," is a guiding principle that underscores the importance of avoiding unnecessary or overly aggressive treatments that could potentially harm the patient.

Autonomy is respected by ensuring that patients are active participants in their care decisions.

This involves not only providing comprehensive information but also respecting patients' choices and preferences, even if they decide against undergoing a procedure. Justice, in the context of cosmetic injections, pertains to providing fair and equitable treatment to all patients, regardless of their background or circumstances.

Practitioners must avoid any form of discrimination and ensure that all patients have access to the information and care they need.

Legal aspects of cosmetic injections are governed by regulations and licensing requirements that vary by region. Practitioners must be thoroughly familiar with the laws and regulations that apply to their practice to ensure compliance.

This includes understanding the scope of practice for different healthcare professionals, as defined by licensing bodies and regulatory agencies. In many jurisdictions, only licensed medical professionals, such as doctors, nurses, and physician assistants, are authorized to perform cosmetic injections.

These professionals must maintain their licenses in good standing, which often requires ongoing education and training to stay current with advances in the field.

Regulations also cover the use of specific substances and devices in cosmetic injections. Only approved products, such as FDA-approved dermal fillers and botulinum toxins, should be used in practice. Practitioners must follow strict guidelines regarding the storage, handling, and administration of these products to ensure their safety and efficacy.

Additionally, proper documentation and record-keeping are essential for legal compliance and for tracking patient outcomes and any adverse events that may occur.

Professional conduct and standards are integral to ethical and legal practice in cosmetic injections. Practitioners must adhere to the codes of conduct established by their professional organizations and regulatory bodies. These codes outline the expected standards of behavior, including maintaining professional boundaries, avoiding conflicts of interest, and practicing with honesty and integrity.

Practitioners should engage in continuous professional development to enhance their skills and knowledge, ensuring that they provide the highest quality of care to their patients.

Continuing education is particularly important in the rapidly evolving field of cosmetic injections. New techniques, products, and technologies are constantly being developed, and staying informed about these advancements is crucial for maintaining a high standard of care. Practitioners should seek out reputable training programs and professional development opportunities to expand their expertise and keep up with the latest best practices.

In addition to clinical skills, effective communication is a key component of professional conduct in cosmetic injections. Practitioners must be able to communicate clearly and empathetically with their patients, explaining procedures and managing expectations.

This includes being honest about what can and cannot be achieved with cosmetic injections, setting realistic goals, and discussing potential risks and complications. Transparent communication helps build trust and fosters a positive patient-practitioner relationship.

Practitioners must also be aware of the psychological aspects of cosmetic procedures. Understanding the motivations and expectations of patients seeking cosmetic injections is essential for providing appropriate care.

Some patients may have unrealistic expectations or underlying psychological issues, such as body dysmorphic disorder, that need to be addressed. In such cases, a referral to a mental health professional may be necessary before proceeding with treatment.

The ethical and legal landscape of cosmetic injections requires a comprehensive understanding of patient rights and responsibilities, adherence to ethical principles, compliance with legal regulations, and commitment to professional conduct and standards. By upholding these principles, practitioners can provide safe, effective, and ethical care to their patients, ensuring positive outcomes and maintaining trust in the field of aesthetic medicine.

CHAPTER 9
Case Studies And Success Stories

Case studies and success stories offer valuable insights into the practical application and outcomes of cosmetic injections. These narratives not only highlight the benefits and transformative effects of various procedures but also provide a detailed understanding of the complexities involved in achieving successful results.

By examining real-life cases, patient testimonials, and lessons learned from challenging scenarios, one can gain a comprehensive view of the effectiveness and nuances of cosmetic injections.

Real-life cases and successful outcomes are a testament to the advancements and capabilities of modern cosmetic injection techniques. These cases often involve a variety of procedures, including dermal fillers, Botox, and fat grafting, each tailored to address specific patient concerns such as facial rejuvenation, volume restoration, and wrinkle reduction.

For instance, a patient seeking to reduce the appearance of deep nasolabial folds might undergo a series of hyaluronic acid filler injections. The procedure, typically completed within a short session, can result in immediate visible improvement, with the patient experiencing a smoother, more youthful contour in the mid-face region. Such successful outcomes not only enhance the patient's aesthetic appearance but also significantly boost their self-esteem and confidence.

In another example, a patient with asymmetrical facial features due to volume loss might benefit from autologous fat grafting. This procedure involves harvesting fat from a donor site on the patient's body, processing it, and then carefully injecting it into the areas needing enhancement. The dual benefit of body contouring from fat removal and facial rejuvenation from fat grafting is a significant advantage.

Success stories from such procedures often highlight the natural-looking results and the long-term durability of the fat grafts, with many patients reporting satisfaction years after the initial treatment. These real-life examples underscore the effectiveness of cosmetic injections in achieving desirable aesthetic results.

Patient testimonials and feedback play a crucial role in understanding the patient experience and satisfaction levels associated with cosmetic injections.

Testimonials often reveal the emotional and psychological impact of the procedures, providing a more holistic view of the outcomes. For instance, a patient undergoing Botox injections for chronic migraines might share their journey, detailing how the procedure not only alleviated their pain but also improved their quality of life by reducing the frequency and severity of their headaches. Such feedback highlights the therapeutic benefits of cosmetic injections beyond aesthetic enhancement.

Another patient might provide a testimonial about their experience with lip augmentation using dermal fillers. Their narrative could emphasize the precision and skill of the injector, the minimal discomfort during the procedure, and the natural-looking enhancement achieved.

These testimonials often include before-and-after photos, showcasing the dramatic improvements and providing visual evidence of the effectiveness of the treatments. The positive feedback from these patients can serve as a powerful endorsement, encouraging others to consider cosmetic injections as a viable solution for their aesthetic concerns.

Lessons learned from challenging cases are invaluable for practitioners seeking to refine their techniques and improve patient outcomes.

These cases often involve complications or less-than-ideal results, providing a learning opportunity to understand the potential pitfalls and how to avoid them.

For instance, a challenging case might involve a patient who experienced asymmetry after a filler injection due to uneven product distribution.

By carefully analyzing the case, the practitioner can identify the factors that led to the issue, such as improper injection technique or inadequate patient assessment, and implement strategies to prevent similar occurrences in the future.

Another example of a challenging case could involve a patient who developed an adverse reaction to a particular injectable product. Through meticulous investigation, the practitioner might determine that the reaction was due to an allergic response or a sensitivity to a component in the product.

This experience underscores the importance of thorough patient screening and the need for practitioners to be knowledgeable about the ingredients and potential side effects of the products they use.

By learning from these challenges, practitioners can enhance their skills, improve patient safety, and achieve more consistent and satisfactory outcomes.

Real-life cases and successful outcomes, patient testimonials, and lessons learned from challenging cases collectively contribute to a deeper understanding of the field of cosmetic injections. These narratives provide concrete examples of the procedures' effectiveness, offer insights into the patient experience, and highlight the importance of continuous learning and improvement in achieving optimal results. Through these stories, both practitioners and patients can appreciate the transformative power of cosmetic injections and the dedication required to master this intricate and ever-evolving field.

Conclusion

Cosmetic injections have transformed the field of aesthetic procedures, offering a range of solutions from enhancing facial symmetry to rejuvenating the skin. With a rich history and continuous evolution, these techniques have become vital in achieving natural-looking, individualized results. Understanding the aesthetic principles behind cosmetic injections, such as facial proportions and artistic techniques, allows practitioners to customize treatments and combine methods for optimal outcomes.

Various types of cosmetic injections, including botulinum toxin, dermal fillers, fat transfer, and platelet-rich plasma (PRP) injections, cater to different needs and preferences. The choice of injection depends on the desired effect, whether it's reducing wrinkles, adding volume, or improving skin texture. Precise knowledge of anatomy and injection techniques, whether using needles or cannulas, ensures that treatments are both effective and safe. Practitioners must master the depth of injection, product distribution, and patient comfort to deliver the best results.

Preparation and patient assessment are crucial steps in the injection process. A thorough consultation, medical history review, and informed consent process lay the foundation for successful treatments. Pre-procedure protocols and guidelines ensure that both patient and practitioner are well-prepared.

Post-procedure care is essential to manage common reactions and prevent complications. Immediate protocols, coupled with vigilant follow-up and monitoring, help maintain the desired outcomes and address any issues promptly. Advanced techniques and innovations, such as combination treatments and the integration of new technologies, continually push the boundaries of what can be achieved with cosmetic injections.

Ethical and legal considerations are paramount in the practice of cosmetic injections. Practitioners must adhere to regulations, maintain professional standards, and prioritize patient rights and responsibilities. Ethical conduct ensures trust and safety in aesthetic practices.

Real-life case studies and patient testimonials highlight the transformative power of cosmetic injections. These success stories not only demonstrate the efficacy of the treatments but also provide valuable lessons from challenging cases. They serve as a testament to the skill and artistry required to achieve excellent results in cosmetic injections.

Cosmetic injections represent a blend of science and art, requiring meticulous technique, continuous learning, and a deep understanding of aesthetic principles.

As innovations continue to emerge, the future of cosmetic injections promises even more advanced and personalized treatments, ensuring that patients can achieve their aesthetic goals with confidence and satisfaction.

www.ingramcontent.com/pod-product-compliance
Lightning Source LLC
Chambersburg PA
CBHW051706250726
48653CB00007B/2874